Ketogenic Breakfast

Recipes

Effective Low-Carb Recipes To Balance Hormones And Effortlessly Reach Your Weight Loss Goal.

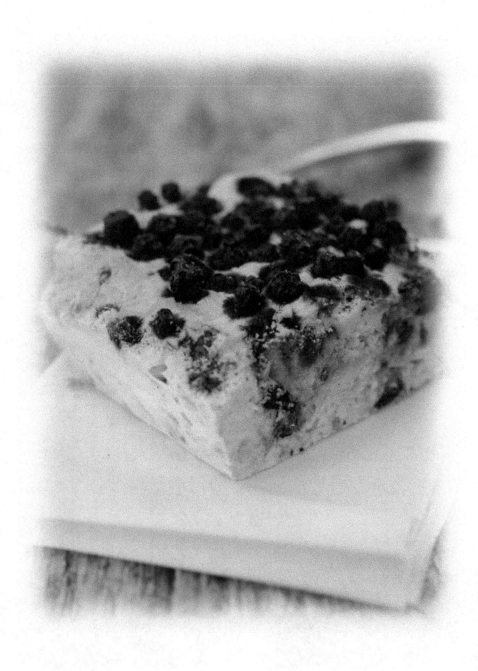

Introduction

Do you want to make a change in your life? Do you want to become a healthier person who can enjoy a new and improved life? Then, you are definitely in the right place. You are about to discover a wonderful and very healthy diet that has changed millions of lives. We are talking about the Ketogenic diet, a lifestyle that will mesmerize you and that will make you a new person in no time.

So, let's sit back, relax and find out more about the Ketogenic diet.

A keto diet is a low carb one. This is the first and one of the most important things you should now. During such a diet, your body makes ketones in your liver and these are used as energy.

Your body will produce less insulin and glucose and a state of ketosis is induced. Ketosis is a natural process that appears when our food intake is lower than usual. The body will soon adapt to this state and therefore you will be able to lose weight in no time but you will also become healthier and your physical and mental performances will improve.

Your blood sugar levels will improve and you won't be predisposed to diabetes. Also, epilepsy and heart diseases can be prevented if you are on a Ketogenic diet.
Your cholesterol will improve and you will feel amazing in no time.

How does that sound?

A Ketogenic diet is simple and easy to follow as long as you follow some simple rules. You don't need to make huge changes but there are some things you should know.
So, here goes!

Now let's start our magical culinary journey!

Ketogenic lifestyle...here we come!

Enjoy!

Avocado Muffins

If you like avocado recipes, then you should really try this next one soon!

Preparation time: 10 minutes **Cooking time:** 20 minutes **Servings:** 12

Ingredients:

- 4 eggs
- 6 bacon slices, chopped
- 1 yellow onion, chopped
- 1 cup coconut milk
- 2 cups avocado, pitted, peeled and chopped
- Salt and black pepper to the taste
- ½ teaspoon baking soda
- ½ cup coconut flour

Directions:

1. Heat up a pan over medium heat, add onion and bacon, stir and brown for a few minutes.
2. In a bowl, mash avocado pieces with a fork and whisk well with the eggs.
3. Add milk, salt, pepper, baking soda and coconut flour and stir everything.
4. Add bacon mix and stir again.
5. Grease a muffin tray with the coconut oil, divide eggs and avocado mix into the tray, introduce in the oven at 350 degrees F and bake for 20 minutes.
6. Divide muffins between plates and serve them for breakfast.

Enjoy!

Nutrition: calories 200, fat 7, fiber 4, carbs 7, protein 5

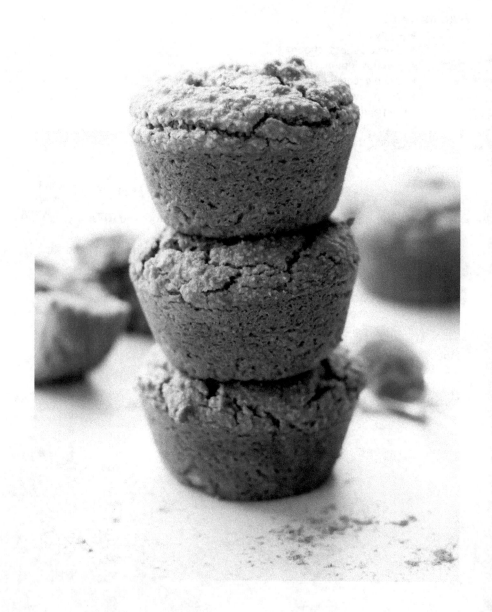

Bacon And Lemon Breakfast Muffins

We are sure you've never tried something like this before! It's a perfect keto breakfast!

Preparation time: 10 minutes **Cooking time:** 20 minutes **Servings:** 12

Ingredients:

- 1 cup bacon, finely chopped
- Salt and black pepper to the taste
- ½ cup ghee, melted
- 3 cups almond flour
- 1 teaspoon baking soda
- 4 eggs
- 2 teaspoons lemon thyme

Directions:

1. In a bowl, mix flour with baking soda and eggs and stir well.
2. Add ghee, lemon thyme, bacon, salt and pepper and whisk well.
3. Divide this into a lined muffin pan, introduce in the oven at 350 degrees F and bake for 20 minutes.
4. Leave muffins to cool down a bit, divide between plates and serve them.

Enjoy!

Nutrition: calories 213, fat 7, fiber 2, carbs 9, protein 8

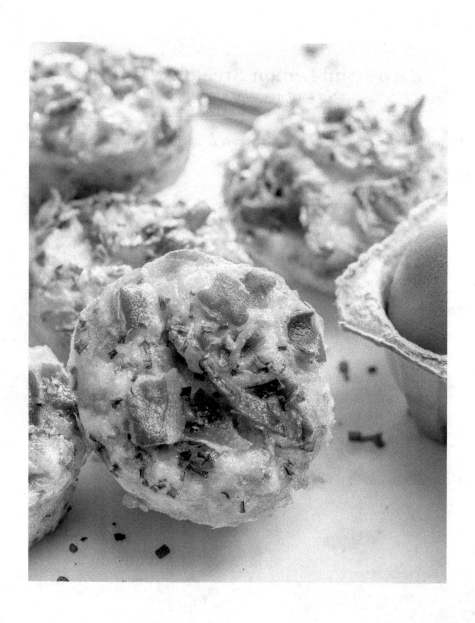

Cheese And Oregano Muffins

We will make you love keto muffins from now on!

Preparation time: 10 minutes **Cooking time:** 25 minutes **Servings:** 6

Ingredients:

- 2 tablespoons olive oil
- 1 egg
- 2 tablespoons parmesan cheese
- ½ teaspoon oregano, dried
- 1 cup almond flour
- ¼ teaspoon baking soda
- Salt and black pepper to the taste
- ½ cup coconut milk
- 1 cup cheddar cheese, grated

Directions:

1. In a bowl, mix flour with oregano, salt, pepper, parmesan and baking soda and stir.
2. In another bowl, mix coconut milk with egg and olive oil and stir well.
3. Combine the 2 mixtures and whisk well.
4. Add cheddar cheese, stir, pour this a lined muffin tray, introduce in the oven at 350 degrees F for 25 minutes.
5. Leave your muffins to cool down for a few minutes, divide them between plates and serve.

Enjoy!

Nutrition: calories 160, fat 3, fiber 2, carbs 6, protein 10

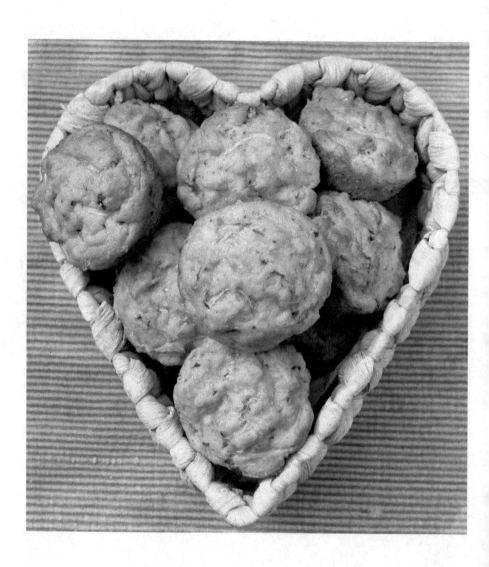

Delicious Turkey Breakfast

Try a Ketogenic turkey breakfast for a change!

Preparation time: 10 minutes **Cooking time:** 20 minutes **Servings:** 1

Ingredients:
- 2 avocado slices
- Salt and black pepper
- 2 bacon sliced
- 2 turkey breast slices, already cooked
- 2 tablespoons coconut oil
- 2 eggs, whisked

Directions:
1. Heat up a pan over medium heat, add bacon slices and brown them for a few minutes.
2. Meanwhile, heat up another pan with the oil over medium heat, add eggs, salt and pepper and scramble them.
3. Divide turkey breast slices on 2 plates.
4. Divide scrambled eggs on each.
5. Divide bacon slices and avocado slices as well and serve.

Enjoy!

Nutrition: calories 135, fat 7, fiber 2, carbs 4, protein 10

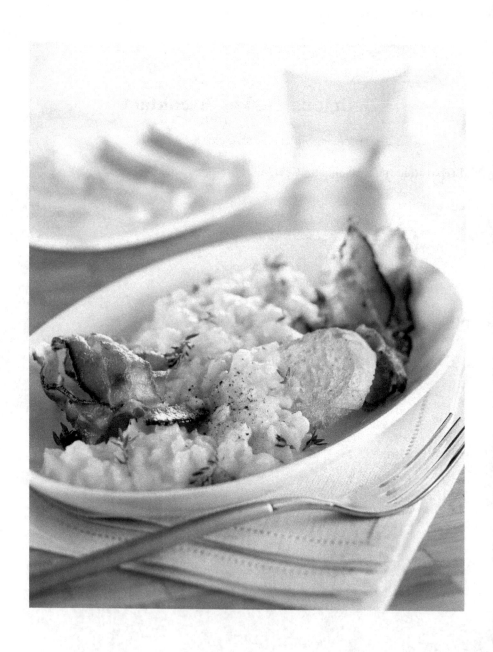

Amazing Burrito

Can you have a burrito for breakfast? Of course, you can!

Preparation time: 10 minutes **Cooking time:** 16 minutes **Servings:** 1

Ingredients:

- 1 teaspoon coconut oil
- 1 teaspoon garlic powder
- 1 teaspoon cumin, ground
- ¼ pound beef meat, ground
- 1 teaspoon sweet paprika
- 1 teaspoon onion powder
- 1 small red onion, julienned
- 1 teaspoon cilantro, chopped
- Salt and black pepper to the taste
- 3 eggs

Directions:

1. Heat up a pan over medium heat, add beef and brown for a few minutes.
2. Add salt, pepper, cumin, garlic and onion powder and paprika, stir, cook for 4 minutes more and take off heat.
3. In a bowl, mix eggs with salt and pepper and whisk well.
4. Heat up a pan with the oil over medium heat, add egg, spread evenly and cook for 6 minutes.
5. Transfer your egg burrito to a plate, divide beef mix, add onion and cilantro, roll and serve.

Enjoy!

Nutrition: calories 280, fat 12, fiber 4, carbs 7, protein 14

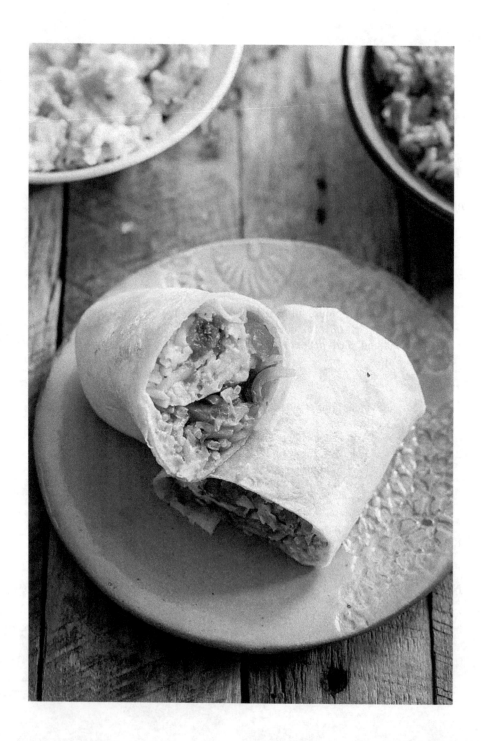

Amazing Breakfast Hash

This breakfast hash is just right for you!

Preparation time: 10 minutes **Cooking time:** 16 minutes **Servings:** 2

Ingredients:
- 1 tablespoon coconut oil
- 2 garlic cloves, minced
- ½ cup beef stock
- Salt and black pepper to the taste
- 1 yellow onion, chopped
- 2 cups corned beef, chopped
- 1 pound radishes, cut in quarters

Directions:
1. Heat up a pan with the oil over medium high heat, add onion, stir and cook for 4 minutes.
2. Add radishes, stir and cook for 5 minutes.
3. Add garlic, stir and cook for 1 minute more.
4. Add stock, beef, salt and pepper, stir, cook for 5 minutes, take off heat and serve.

Enjoy!

Nutrition: calories 240, fat 7, fiber 3, carbs 12, protein 8

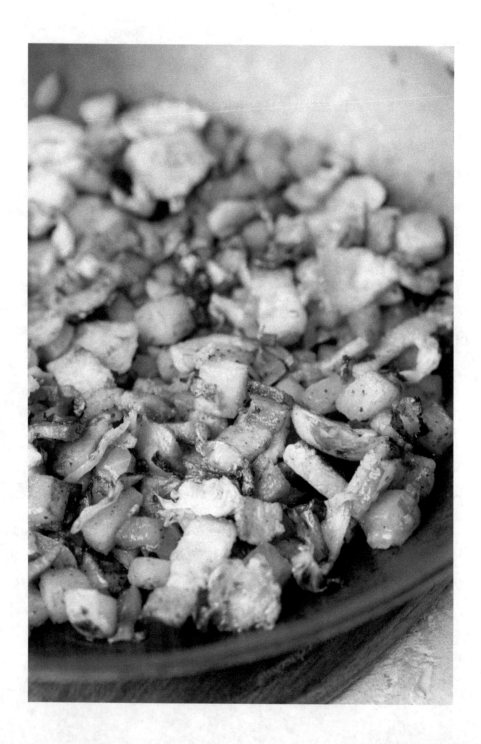

Brussels Sprouts Delight

This is so tasty and very easy to make! It's a great keto breakfast idea for you!

Preparation time: 10 minutes **Cooking time:** 12 minutes **Servings:** 3

Ingredients:

- 3 eggs
- Salt and black pepper to the taste
- 1 tablespoon ghee, melted
- 2 shallots, minced
- 2 garlic cloves, minced
- 12 ounces Brussels sprouts, thinly sliced
- 2 ounces bacon, chopped
- 1 and ½ tablespoons apple cider vinegar

Directions:

1. Heat up a pan over medium heat, add bacon, stir, cook until it's crispy, transfer to a plate and leave aside for now.
2. Heat up the pan again over medium heat, add shallots and garlic, stir and cook for 30 seconds.
3. Add Brussels sprouts, salt, pepper and apple cider vinegar, stir and cook for 5 minutes.
4. Return bacon to pan, stir and cook for 5 minutes more.
5. Add ghee, stir and make a hole in the center.
6. Crack eggs into the pan, cook until they are done and serve right away.

Enjoy!

Nutrition: calories 240, fat 7, fiber 4, carbs 7, protein 12

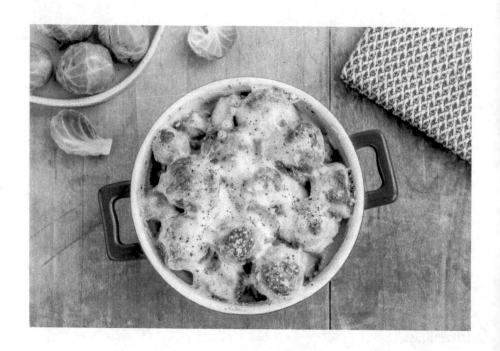

Breakfast Cereal Nibs

Pay attention and learn how to prepare the best keto cereal nibs!

Preparation time: 10 minutes **Cooking time:** 45minutes **Servings:** 4

Ingredients:
- 4 tablespoons hemp hearts
- ½ cup chia seeds
- 1 cup water
- 1 tablespoon vanilla extract
- 1 tablespoon psyllium powder
- 2 tablespoons coconut oil
- 1 tablespoon swerve
- 2 tablespoons cocoa nibs

Directions:
1. In a bowl, mix chia seeds with water, stir and leave aside for 5 minutes.
2. Add hemp hearts, vanilla extract, psyllium powder, oil and swerve and stir well with your mixer.
3. Add cocoa nibs, and stir until you obtain a dough.
4. Divide dough into 2 pieces, shape into cylinder form, place on a lined baking sheet, flatten well, cover with a parchment paper, introduce in the oven at 285 degrees F and bake for 20 minutes.
5. Remove the parchment paper and bake for 25 minutes more.
6. Take cylinders out of the oven, leave aside to cool down and cut into small pieces.
7. Serve in the morning with some almond milk.

Enjoy!

Nutrition: calories 245, fat 12, fiber 12, carbs 2, protein 9

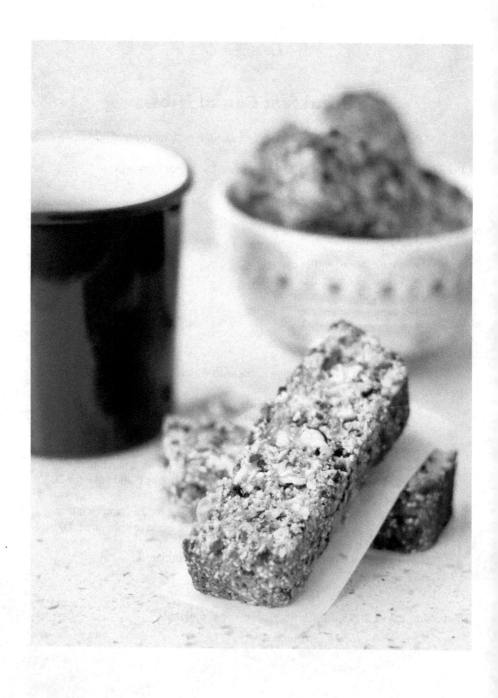

Breakfast Chia Pudding

Try a chia pudding this morning!

Preparation time: 10 minutes **Cooking time:** 30 minutes **Servings:** 2

Ingredients:

- 2 tablespoons coffee
- 2 cups water
- 1/3 cup chia seeds
- 1 tablespoon swerve
- 1 tablespoon vanilla extract
- 2 tablespoons cocoa nibs
- 1/3 cup coconut cream

Directions:

1. Heat up a small pot with the water over medium heat, bring to a boil, add coffee, simmer for 15 minutes, take off heat and strain into a bowl.
2. Add vanilla extract, coconut cream, swerve, cocoa nibs andchia seeds, stir well, keep in the fridge for 30 minutes, divide into 2 breakfast bowls and serve.

Enjoy!

Nutrition: calories 100, fat 0.4, fiber 4, carbs 3, protein 3

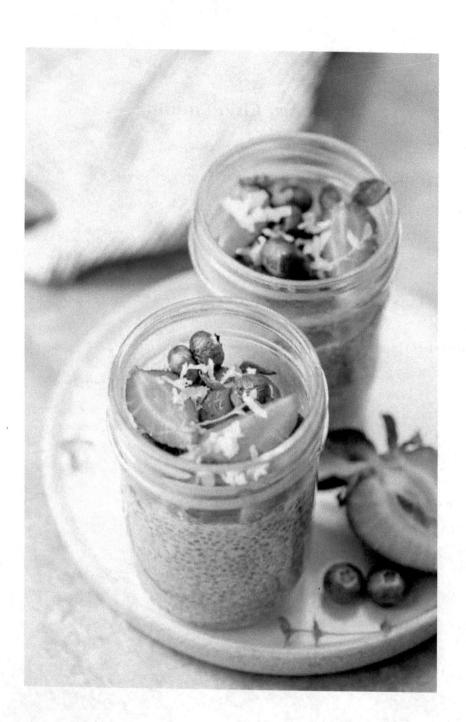

Delicious Hemp Porridge

It's a hearty and 100% keto breakfast idea!

Preparation time: 3 minutes **Cooking time:** 3 minutes **Servings:** 1

Ingredients:
- 1 tablespoon chia seeds
- 1 cup almond milk
- 2 tablespoons flax seeds
- ½ cup hemp hearts
- ½ teaspoon cinnamon, ground
- 1 tablespoon stevia
- ¾ teaspoon vanilla extract
- ¼ cup almond flour
- 1 tablespoon hemp hearts for serving

Directions:
1. In a pan, mix almond milk with ½ cup hemp hearts, chia seeds, stevia, flax seeds, cinnamon and vanilla extract, stir well and heat up over medium heat.
2. Cook for 2 minutes, take off heat, add almond flour, stir well and pour into a bowl.
3. Top with 1 tablespoon hemp hearts and serve.

Enjoy!

Nutrition: calories 230, fat 12, fiber 7, carbs 3, protein 43

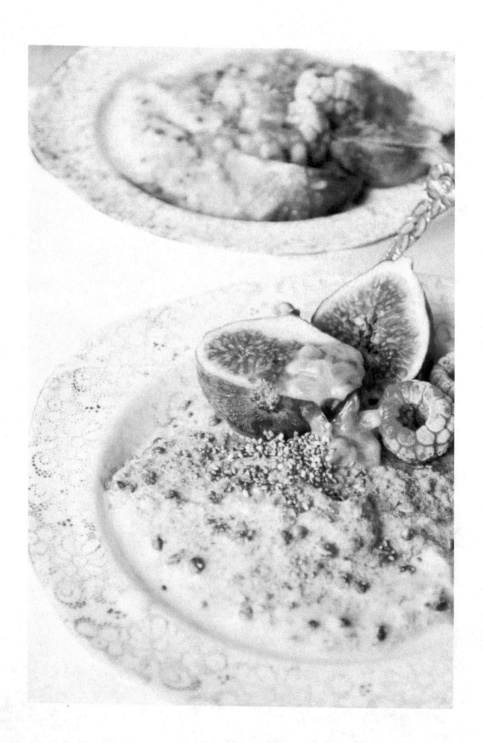

Simple Breakfast Cereal

It's so easy to make a tasty keto breakfast!

Preparation time: 10 minutes **Cooking time:** 3 minutes **Servings:** 2

Ingredients:
- ½ cup coconut, shredded
- 4 teaspoons ghee
- 2 cups almond milk
- 1 tablespoon stevia
- A pinch of salt
- 1/3 cup macadamia nuts, chopped
- 1/3 cup walnuts, chopped
- 1/3 cup flax seed

Directions:
1. Heat up a pot with the ghee over medium heat, add milk, coconut, salt, macadamia nuts, walnuts, flax seed and stevia and stir well.
2. Cook for 3 minutes, stir again, take off heat and leave aside for 10 minutes.
3. Divide into 2 bowls and serve.

Enjoy!

Nutrition: calories 140, fat 3, fiber 2, carbs 1.5, protein 7

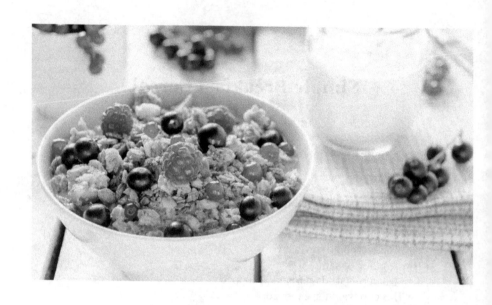

Simple Egg Porridge

It's so simple and tasty!

Preparation time: 10 minutes **Cooking time:** 4 minutes **Servings:** 2

Ingredients:
- 2 eggs
- 1 tablespoon stevia
- 1/3 cup heavy cream
- 2 tablespoons ghee, melted
- A pinch of cinnamon, ground

Directions:
1. In a bowl, mix eggs with stevia and heavy cream and whisk well.
2. Heat up a pan with the ghee over medium high heat, add egg mix and cook until they are done.
3. Transfer to 2 bowls, sprinkle cinnamon on top and serve.

Enjoy!

Nutrition: calories 340, fat 12, fiber 10, carbs 3, protein 14

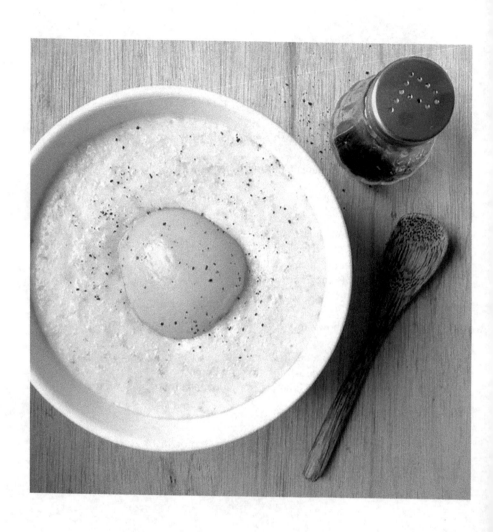

Delicious Pancakes

Why don't you try these delicious keto pancakes today?

Preparation time: 3 minutes **Cooking time:** 12 minutes **Servings:** 4

Ingredients:

- ½ teaspoon cinnamon, ground
- 1 teaspoon stevia
- 2 eggs
- Cooking spray
- 2 ounces cream cheese

Directions:

1. In your blender, mix eggs with cream cheese, stevia and cinnamon and blend well.
2. Heat up a pan with some cooking spray over medium high heat, pour ¼ of the batter, spread well, cook for 2 minutes, flip and cook for 1 minute more.
3. Transfer to a plate and repeat the action with the rest of the batter.
4. Serve them right away.

Enjoy!

Nutrition: calories 344, fat 23, fiber 12, carbs 3, protein 16

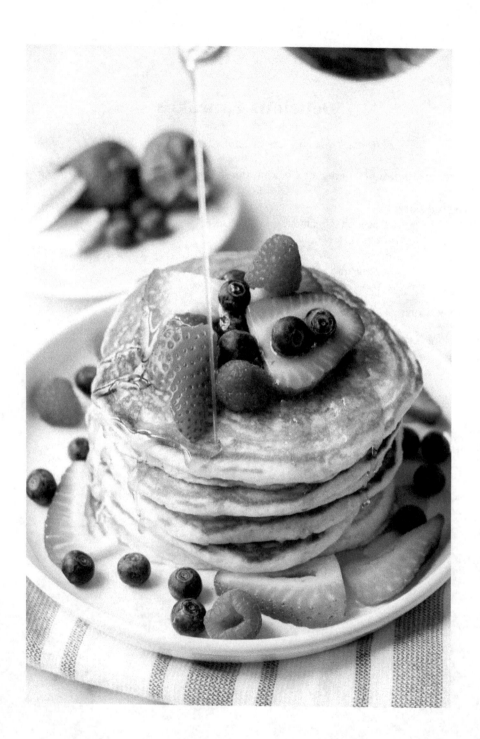

Almond Pancakes

These are so delicious! Try them!

Preparation time: 10 minutes **Cooking time:** 10 minutes **Servings:** 12

Ingredients:

- 6 eggs
- A pinch of salt
- ½ cup coconut flour
- ¼ cup stevia
- 1/3 cup coconut, shredded
- ½ teaspoon baking powder
- 1 cup almond milk
- ¼ cup coconut oil
- 1 teaspoon almond extract
- ¼ cup almonds, toasted
- 2 ounces cocoa chocolate
- Cooking spray

Directions:

1. In a bowl, mix coconut flour with stevia, salt, baking powder and coconut and stir.
2. Add coconut oil, eggs, almond milk and the almond extract and stir well again.
3. Add chocolate and almonds and whisk well again.
4. Heat up a pan with cooking spray over medium heat, add 2 tablespoons batter, spread into a circle, cook until it's golden, flip, cook again until it's done and transfer to a pan.
5. Repeat with the rest of the batter and serve your pancakes right away.

Enjoy!

Nutrition: calories 266, fat 13, fiber 8, carbs 10, protein 11

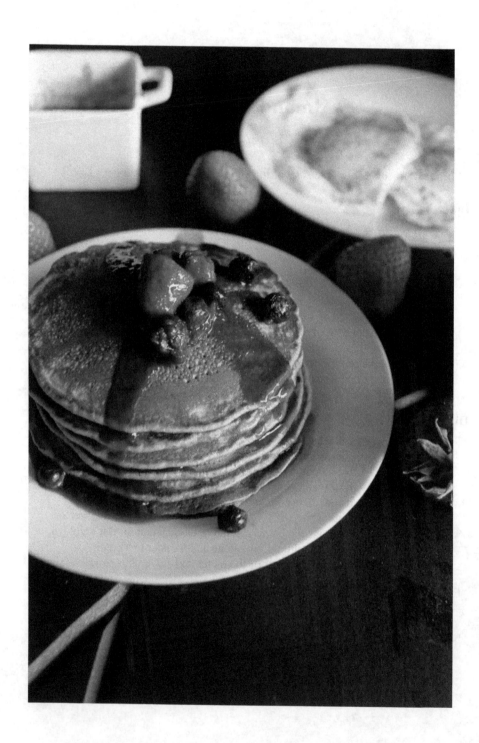

Delicious Pumpkin Pancakes

These keto pumpkin pancakes will make your day!

Preparation time: 10 minutes **Cooking time:** 15 minutes **Servings:** 6

Ingredients:

- 1 ounce egg white protein
- 2 ounces hazelnut flour
- 2 ounces flax seeds, ground
- 1 teaspoon baking powder
- 1 cup coconut cream
- 1 tablespoon chai masala
- 1 teaspoon vanilla extract
- ½ cup pumpkin puree
- 3 eggs
- 5 drops stevia
- 1 tablespoon swerve
- 1 teaspoon coconut oil

Directions:

1. In a bowl, mix flax seeds with hazelnut flour, egg white protein, baking powder and chai masala and stir.
2. In another bowl, mix coconut cream with vanilla extract, pumpkin puree, eggs, stevia and swerve and stir well.
3. Combine the 2 mixtures and stir well.
4. Heat up a pan with the oil over medium high heat, pour 1/6 of the batter, spread into a circle, cover, reduce heat to low, cook for 3 minutes on each side and transfer to a plate.
5. Repeat with the rest of the batter and serve your pumpkin pancakes right away.

Enjoy!

Nutrition: calories 400, fat 23, fiber 4, carbs 5, protein 21

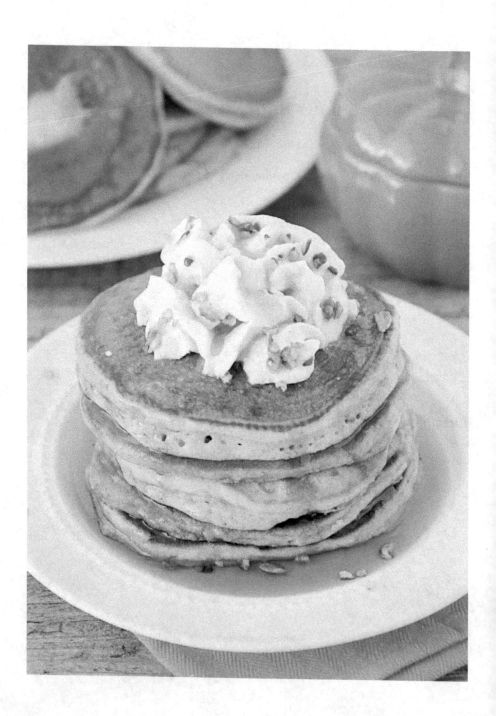

Simple Breakfast French Toast

Believe it or not, this is a keto breakfast!

Preparation time: 5 minutes **Cooking time:** 45 minutes **Servings:** 18

Ingredients:
- 1 cup whey protein
- 12 egg whites
- 4 ounces cream cheese

For the French toast:
- 1 teaspoon vanilla
- ½ cup coconut milk
- 2 eggs
- 1 teaspoon cinnamon, ground
- ½ cup ghee, melted
- ½ cup almond milk
- ½ cup swerve

Directions:
1. In a bowl, mix 12 egg whites with your mixer for a few minutes.
2. Add protein and stir gently.
3. Add cream cheese and stir again.
4. Pour this into 2 greased bread pans, introduce in the oven at 325 degrees F and bake for 45 minutes.
5. Leave breads to cool down and slice them into 18 pieces.
6. In a bowl, mix 2 eggs with vanilla, cinnamon and coconut milk and whisk well.
7. Dip bread slices in this mix.
8. Heat up a pan with some coconut oil over medium heat, add bread slices, cook until they are golden on each side and divide between plates.
9. Heat up a pan with the ghee over high heat, add almond milk and heat up well.
10. Add swerve, stir and take off heat.
11. Leave aside to cool down a bit and drizzle over French toasts.

Enjoy!

Nutrition: calories 200, fat 12, fiber 1, carbs 1, protein 7

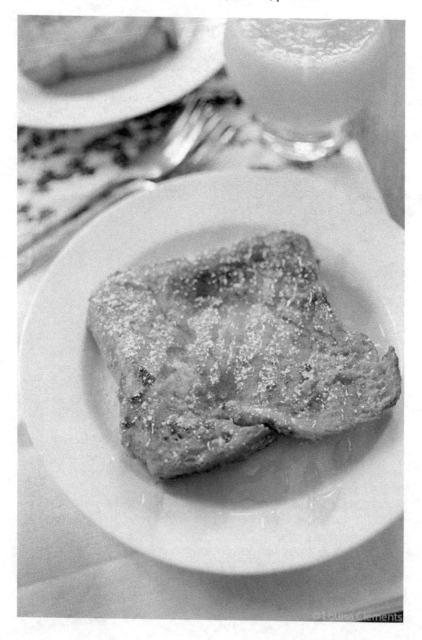

Amazing Waffles

Get ready for a really tasty breakfast!

Preparation time: 10 minutes **Cooking time:** 20 minutes **Servings:** 5

Ingredients:

- 5 eggs, separated
- 3 tablespoons almond milk
- 1 teaspoon baking powder
- 3 tablespoons stevia
- 4 tablespoons coconut flour
- 2 teaspoon vanilla
- 4 ounces ghee, melted

Directions:

1. In a bowl, whisk egg white using your mixer.
2. In another bowl mix flour with stevia, baking powder and egg yolks and whisk well.
3. Add vanilla, ghee and milk and stir well again.
4. Add egg white and stir gently everything.
5. Pour some of the mix into your waffle maker and cook until it's golden.
6. Repeat with the rest of the batter and serve your waffles right away.

Enjoy!

Nutrition: calories 240, fat 23, fiber 2, carbs 4, protein 7

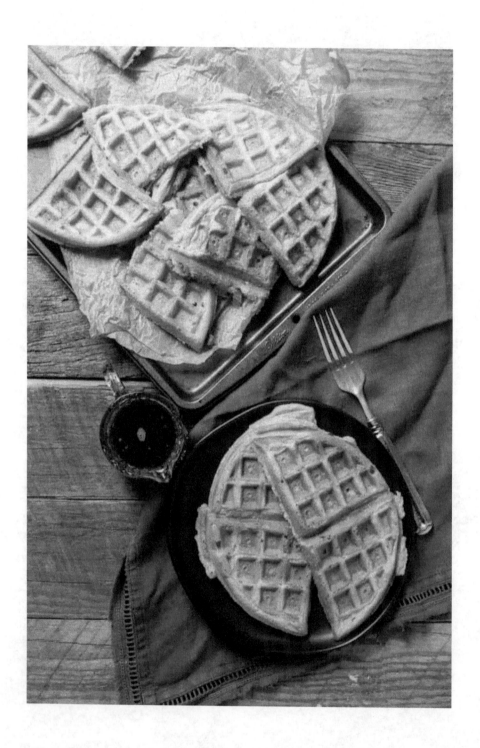

Baked Granola

This is so amazing and tasty! We love it!

Preparation time: 10 minutes **Cooking time:** 60 minutes **Servings:** 4

Ingredients:
- ½ cup almonds, chopped
- 1 cup pecans, chopped
- ½ cup walnuts, chopped
- ½ cup coconut, flaked
- ¼ cup flax meal
- ½ cup almond milk
- ¼ cup sunflower seeds
- ¼ cup pepitas
- ½ cup stevia
- ¼ cup ghee, melted
- 1 teaspoon honey
- 1 teaspoon vanilla
- 1 teaspoon cinnamon, ground
- A pinch of salt
- ½ teaspoon nutmeg
- ¼ cup water

Directions:
1. In a bowl, mix almonds with pecans, walnuts, coconut, flax meal, milk, sunflower seeds, pepitas, stevia, ghee, honey, vanilla, cinnamon, salt, nutmeg and water and whisk very well.
2. Grease a baking sheet with parchment paper, spread granola mix and press well.
3. Cover with another piece of parchment paper, introduce in the oven at 250 degrees F and bake for 1 hour.
4. Take granola out of the oven, leave aside to cool down, break into pieces and serve.

Enjoy!

Nutrition: calories 340, fat 32, fiber 12, carbs 20, protein 20

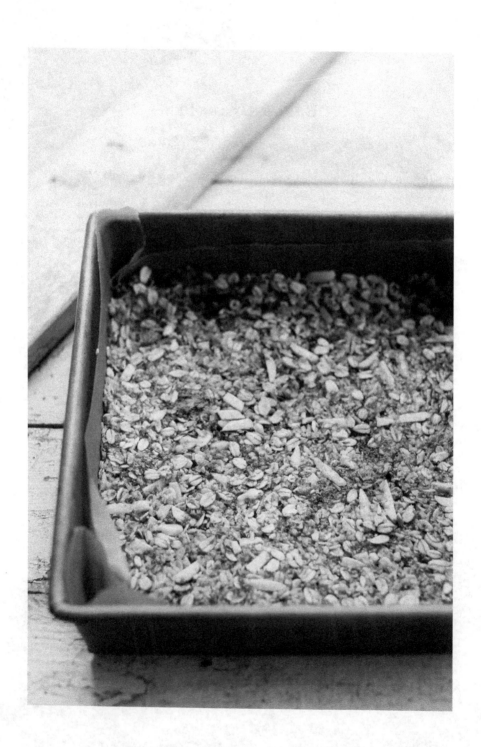

Amazing Smoothie

This smoothie is the best!

Preparation time: 5 minutes **Cooking time:** 0 minutes **Servings:** 1

Ingredients:
- 2 brazil nuts
- 1 cup coconut milk
- 10 almonds
- 2 cups spinach leaves
- 1 teaspoon green powder
- 1 teaspoon whey protein
- 1 tablespoon psyllium seeds
- 1 tablespoon potato starch

Directions:
1. In your blender, mix spinach with brazil nuts, coconut milk and almonds and blend well.
2. Add green powder, whey protein, potato starch and psyllium seeds and blend well again.
3. Pour into a tall glass and consume for breakfast.

Enjoy!

Nutrition: calories 340, fat 30, fiber 7, carbs 7, protein 12

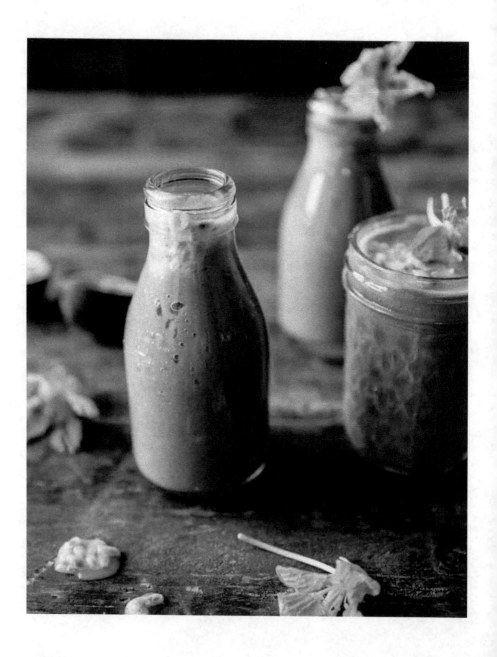

Refreshing Breakfast Smoothie

It's so healthy and fresh! We love it!

Preparation time: 5 minutes **Cooking time:** 0 minutes **Servings:** 6

Ingredients:

- 1 cup lettuce leaves
- 4 cups water
- 2 tablespoons parsley leaves
- 1 tablespoon ginger, grated
- 1 tablespoon swerve
- 1 cup cucumber, sliced
- ½ avocado, pitted and peeled
- ½ cup kiwi, peeled and sliced
- 1/3 cup pineapple, chopped

Directions:

1. In your blender, mix water with lettuce leaves, pineapple, parsley, cucumber, ginger, kiwi, avocado and swerve and blend very well.
2. Pour into glasses and serve for a keto breakfast.

Enjoy!

Nutrition: calories 60, fat 2, fiber 3, carbs 3, protein 1

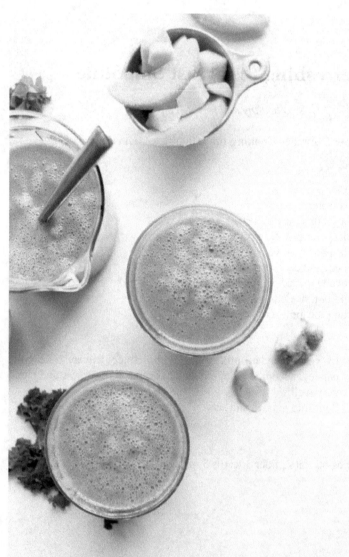

Amazing Breakfast In A Glass

Don't bother making something complex for breakfast! Try this amazing keto drink!

Preparation time: 3 minutes **Cooking time:** 0 minutes **Servings:** 2

Ingredients:
- 10 ounces canned coconut milk
- 1 cup favorite greens
- ¼ cup cocoa nibs
- 1 cup water
- 1 cup cherries, frozen
- ¼ cup cocoa powder
- 1 small avocado, pitted and peeled
- ¼ teaspoon turmeric

Directions:
1. In your blender, mix coconut milk with avocado, cocoa powder, cherries and turmeric and blend well.
2. Add water, greens and cocoa nibs, blend for 2 minutes more, pour into glasses and serve.

Enjoy!

Nutrition: calories 100, fat 3, fiber 2, carbs 3, protein 5

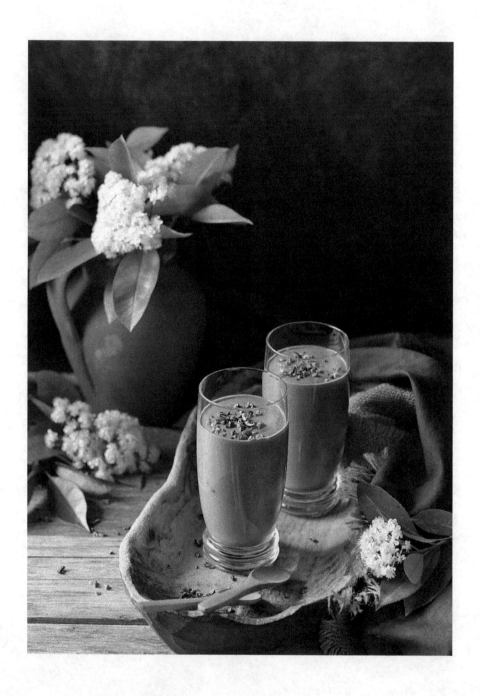

Delicious Chicken Quiche

It's so delicious that you will ask for more!

Preparation time: 10 minutes **Cooking time:** 45 minutes **Servings:** 5

Ingredients:

- 7 eggs
- 2 cups almond flour
- 2 tablespoons coconut oil
- Salt and black pepper to the taste
- 2 zucchinis, grated
- ½ cup heavy cream
- 1 teaspoon fennel seeds
- 1 teaspoon oregano, dried
- 1 pound chicken meat, ground

Directions:

1. In your food processor, blend almond flour with a pinch of salt.
2. Add 1 egg and coconut oil and blend well.
3. Place dough in a greased pie pan and press well on the bottom.
4. Heat up a pan over medium heat, add chicken meat, brown for a couple of minutes, take off heat and leave aside.
5. In a bowl, mix 6 eggs with salt, pepper, oregano, cream and fennel seeds and whisk well.
6. Add chicken meat and stir again.
7. Pour this into pie crust, spread, introduce in the oven at 350 degrees F and bake for 40 minutes.
8. Leave the pie to cool down a bit before slicing and serving it for breakfast!

Enjoy!

Nutrition: calories 300, fat 23, fiber 3, carbs 4, protein 18

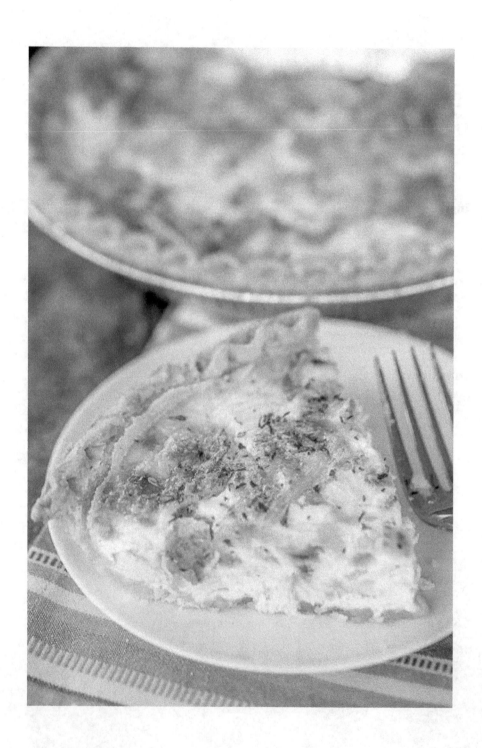

Delicious Steak And Eggs

This is so rich and hearty! Dare and try this for breakfast tomorrow!

Preparation time: 10 minutes **Cooking time:** 10 minutes **Servings:** 1

Ingredients:

- 4 ounces sirloin
- 1 small avocado, pitted, peeled and sliced
- 3 eggs
- 1 tablespoon ghee
- Salt and black pepper to the taste

Directions:

1. Heat up a pan with the ghee over medium high heat, crack eggs into the pan and cook them as you wish.
2. Season with salt and pepper, take off heat and transfer to a plate.
3. Heat up another pan over medium high heat, add sirloin, cook for 4 minutes, take off heat, leave aside to cool down and cut into thin strips.
4. Season with salt and pepper to the taste and place next to the eggs.
5. Add avocado slices on the side and serve.

Enjoy!

Nutrition: calories 500, fat 34, fiber 10, carbs 3, protein 40

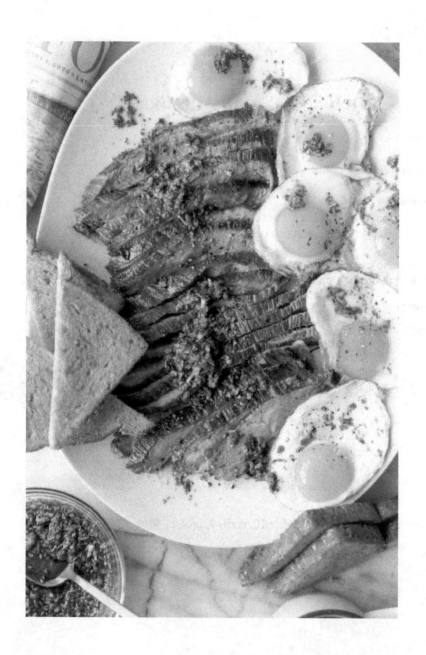

Amazing Chicken Omelet

It tastes amazing and it looks incredible! It's perfect!

Preparation time: 10 minutes **Cooking time:** 10 minutes **Servings:** 1

Ingredients:

- 1 ounce rotisserie chicken, shredded
- 1 teaspoon mustard
- 1 tablespoon homemade mayonnaise
- 1 tomato, chopped
- 2 bacon slices, cooked and crumbled
- 2 eggs
- 1 small avocado, pitted, peeled and chopped
- Salt and black pepper to the taste

Directions:

1. In a bowl, mix eggs with some salt and pepper and whisk gently.
2. Heat up a pan over medium heat, spray with some cooking oil, add eggs and cook your omelet for 5 minutes.
3. Add chicken, avocado, tomato, bacon, mayo and mustard on one half of the omelet.
4. Fold omelet, cover pan and cook for 5 minutes more.
5. Transfer to a plate and serve.

Enjoy!

Nutrition: calories 400, fat 32, fiber 6, carbs 4, protein 25

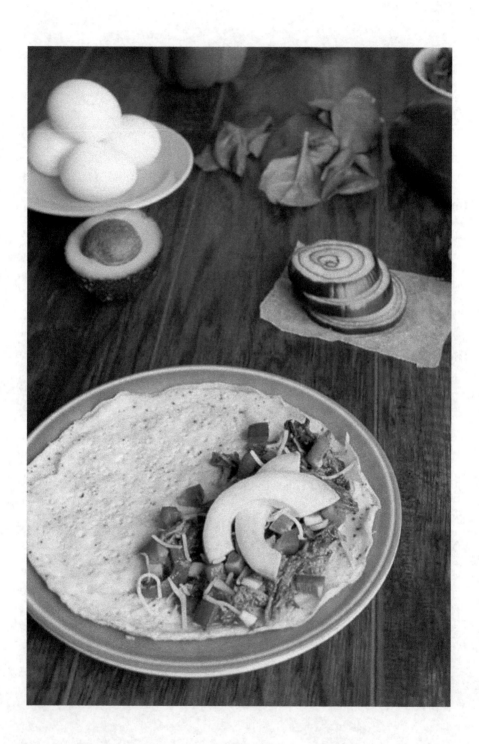

Simple Smoothie Bowl

It's one of the best keto breakfast ideas ever!

Preparation time: 5 minutes **Cooking time:** 0 minutes **Servings:** 1

Ingredients:
- 2 ice cubes
- 1 tablespoon coconut oil
- 2 tablespoons heavy cream
- 1 cup spinach
- ½ cup almond milk
- 1 teaspoon protein powder
- 4 raspberries
- 1 tablespoon coconut ,shredded
- 4 walnuts
- 1 teaspoon chia seeds

Directions:
1. In your blender, mix milk with spinach, cream, ice, protein powder and coconut oil, blend well and transfer to a bowl.
2. Top your bowl with raspberries, coconut, walnuts and chia seeds and serve.

Enjoy!

Nutrition: calories 450, fat 34, fiber 4, carbs 4, protein 35

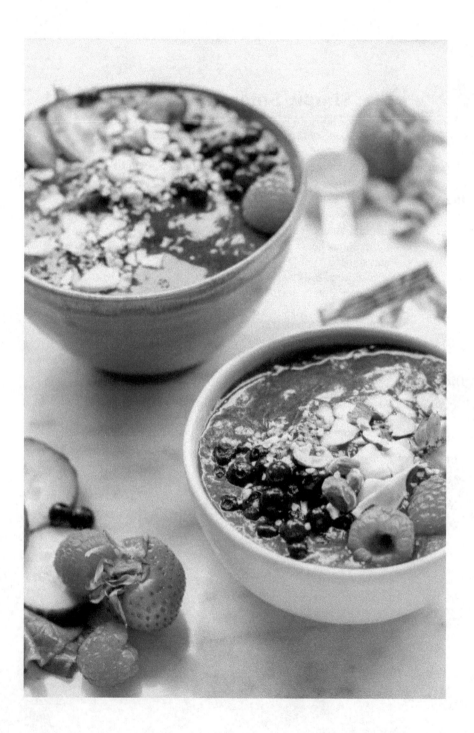

Feta Omelet

The combination of ingredients is just wonderful!

Preparation time: 10 minutes **Cooking time:** 10 minutes **Servings:** 1

Ingredients:
- 3 eggs
- 1 tablespoon ghee
- 1 ounce feta cheese, crumbled
- 1 tablespoon heavy cream
- 1 tablespoon jarred pesto
- Salt and black pepper to the taste

Directions:
1. In a bowl, mix eggs with heavy cream, salt and pepper and whisk well.
2. Heat up a pan with the ghee over medium high heat, add whisked eggs, spread into the pan and cook your omelet until it's fluffy.
3. Sprinkle cheese and spread pesto on your omelet, fold in half, cover pan and cook for 5 minutes more.
4. Transfer omelet to a plate and serve.

Enjoy!

Nutrition: calories 500, fat 43, fiber 6, carbs 3, protein 30

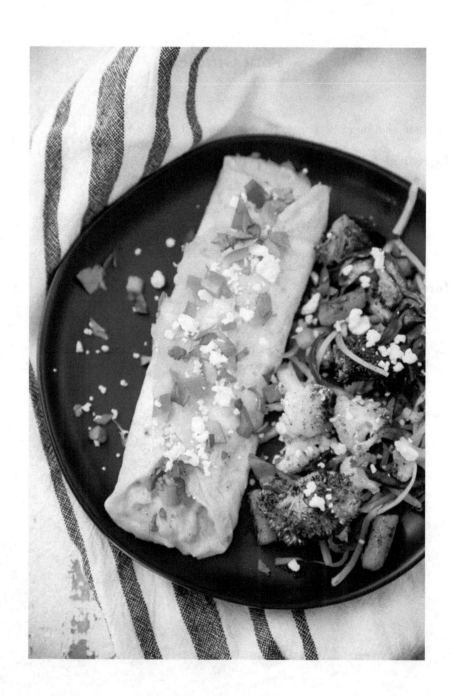

Breakfast Meatloaf

This is something worth trying as soon as possible!

Preparation time: 10 minutes **Cooking time:** 35 minutes **Servings:** 4

Ingredients:
- 1 teaspoon ghee
- 1 small yellow onion, chopped
- 1 pound sweet sausage, chopped
- 6 eggs
- 1 cup cheddar cheese, shredded
- 4 ounces cream cheese, soft
- Salt and black pepper to the taste
- 2 tablespoons scallions, chopped

Directions:
1. In a bowl, mix eggs with salt, pepper, onion, sausage and half of the cream and whisk well.
2. Grease a meatloaf with the ghee, pour sausage and eggs mix, introduce in the oven at 350 degrees F and bake for 30 minutes.
3. Take meatloaf out of the oven, leave aside for a couple of minutes, spread the rest of the cream cheese on top and sprinkle scallions and cheddar cheese all over.
4. Introduce meatloaf in the oven again and bake for 5 minutes more.
5. After the time has passed, broil meatloaf for 3 minutes, leave it aside to cool down a bit, slice and serve it.

Enjoy!

Nutrition: calories 560, fat 32, fiber 1, carbs 6, protein 45

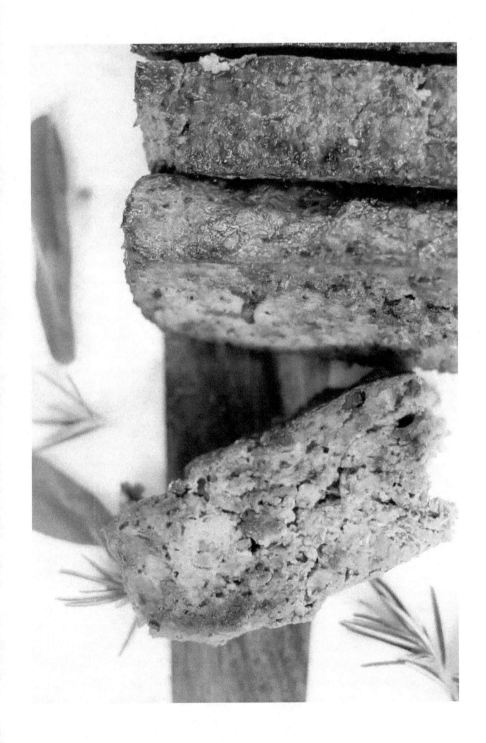

Breakfast Tuna Salad

You will love this Ketogenic breakfast from now on!

Preparation time: 10 minutes **Cooking time:** 0 minutes **Servings:** 4

Ingredients:

- 2 tablespoons sour cream
- 12 ounces tuna in olive oil
- 4 leeks, finely chopped
- Salt and black pepper to the taste
- A pinch of chili flakes
- 1 tablespoon capers
- 8 tablespoons homemade mayonnaise

Directions:

1. In a salad bowl, mix tuna with capers, salt, pepper, leeks, chili flakes, sour cream and mayo.
2. Stir well and serve with some crispy bread.

Enjoy!

Nutrition: calories 160, fat 2, fiber 1, carbs 2, protein 6

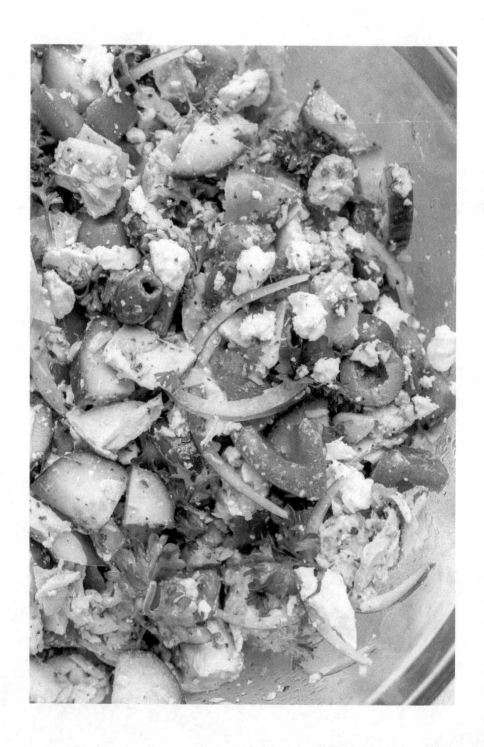

Incredible Breakfast Salad In A Jar

You can even take this at the office!

Preparation time: 10 minutes **Cooking time:** 0 minutes **Servings:** 1

Ingredients:

- 1 ounce favorite greens
- 1 ounce red bell pepper, chopped
- 1 ounce cherry tomatoes, halved
- 4 ounces rotisserie chicken, roughly chopped
- 4 tablespoons extra virgin olive oil
- ½ scallion, chopped
- 1 ounce cucumber, chopped
- Salt and black pepper to the taste

Directions:

1. In a bowl, mix greens with bell pepper, tomatoes, scallion, cucumber, salt, pepper and olive oil and toss to coat well.
2. Transfer this to a jar, top with chicken pieces and serve for breakfast.

Enjoy!

Nutrition: calories 180, fat 12, fiber 4, carbs 5, protein 17

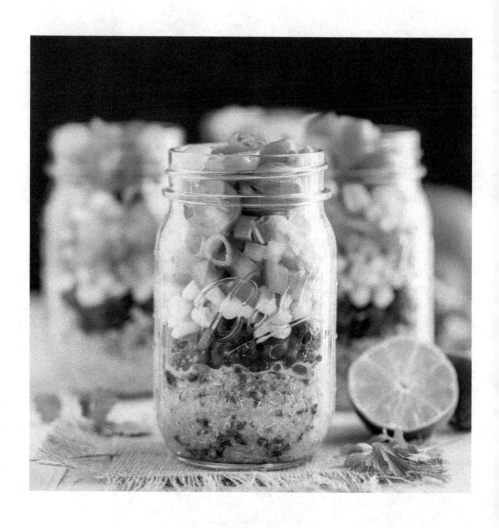

Delicious Naan Bread And Butter

Try this special keto breakfast! It's so easy to make!

Preparation time: 10 minutes **Cooking time:** 10 minutes **Servings:** 6

Ingredients:
- 7 tablespoons coconut oil
- ¾ cup coconut flour
- 2 tablespoons psyllium powder
- ½ teaspoon baking powder
- Salt to the taste
- 2 cups hot water
- Some coconut oil for frying
- 2 garlic cloves, minced
- 3.5 ounces ghee

Directions:
1. In a bowl, mix coconut flour with baking powder, salt and psyllium powder and stir.
2. Add 7 tablespoons coconut oil and the hot water and start kneading your dough.
3. Leave aside for 5 minutes, divide into 6 balls and flatten them on a working surface.
4. Heat up a pan with some coconut oil over medium high heat, add naan breads to the pan, fry them until they are golden and transfer them to a plate.
5. Heat up a pan with the ghee over medium high heat, add garlic, salt and pepper, stir and cook for 2 minutes.
6. Brush naan breads with this mix and pour the rest into a bowl.
7. Serve in the morning.

Enjoy!

Nutrition: calories 140, fat 9, fiber 2, carbs 3, protein 4

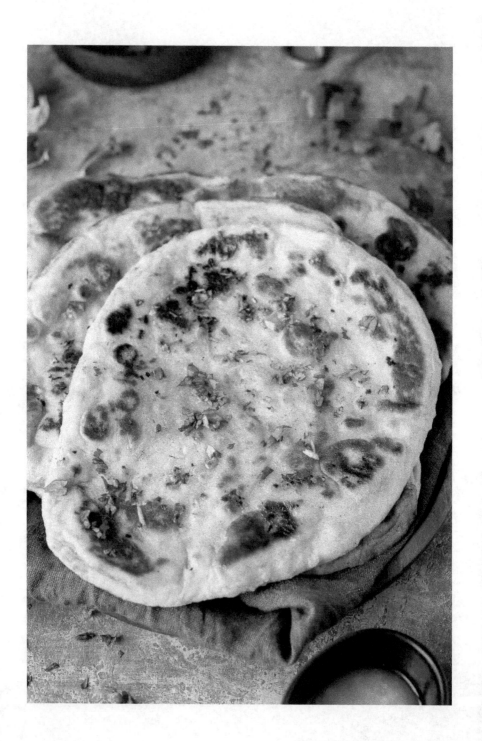

CPSIA information can be obtained
at www.ICGtesting.com
Printed in the USA
LVHW022110110521
687091LV00012B/2691